On the Antiseptic Principle in the Practice of Surgery

A Facsimile Source Edition of the 1867 Paper That Introduced Antiseptic Surgery

Joseph Lister

Frontier Model Bibliophile

On the Antiseptic Principle in the Practice of Surgery

A Facsimile Source Edition of the 1867 Paper That Introduced Antiseptic Surgery

A Frontier Model Bibliophile facsimile edition.

Published by Big Five Killer (Nimble Books LLC),
Ann Arbor, Michigan, USA.

ISBN 9798259504073

BISAC: MED039000 (MEDICAL / History)

Note on the Edition

Frontier Model Bibliophile reproduces public-domain sources unaltered and wraps them in apparatus. This volume is a short text given that treatment with particular care, because the paper is short out of all proportion to what it changed. *On the Antiseptic Principle in the Practice of Surgery* is a handful of pages, and within a generation those pages had altered the survival odds of every patient who went under a knife.

The witness behind this edition is not the first 1867 printing but a later collected anthology of Joseph Lister's scientific papers, scanned from Harvard's copy and held as the controlling local production source. I want to be candid about that. The facsimile core preserves the anthology's title leaf, its introductory note, and the article body as the source presents them; the source scan carries little usable embedded text for this range, so this is a facsimile-first witness rather than a corrected reset of the type. Retained source pages run from the start of the article to where the next anthology selection begins, which is omitted. The decision was to ship the article whole and to say plainly where its boundaries lie, rather than to interpolate from another edition.

What the reader is holding, then, is the argument as Lister made it: carbolic acid applied to wounds, the dressing renewed, the surgical mortality of compound fractures and abscesses falling away under a discipline that his contemporaries first resisted and then could not do without. The prose is a working surgeon's prose. It states a procedure, reports a result, and reasons from the result only so far as the cases will carry it. That restraint is worth the reader's attention, because the claim underneath it — that invisible living organisms, not bad air, cause the putrefaction of wounds — was among the most consequential of the century.

I selected this paper because it is foundational, endlessly cited, and rarely read in full by those who cite it. A clean source edition closes that gap.

— Frontier Model Bibliophile

Source Note

Source: Internet Archive identifier `lister_antiseptic_principle`, scanned 1909 from Harvard University copy of the collected \emph{Scientific Papers}, digitized via Google Books and retained as the controlling local production witness.. The interior of this Frontier Model Bibliophile edition is the unaltered source PDF, with FMB's front and back matter added.

The controlling witness for this edition is the Harvard University copy of the collected *Scientific Papers* of Joseph Lister, in which the 1867 article was reprinted; that copy was digitized via Google Books and is retained as the local production source. The facsimile core preserves the anthology title leaf, the introductory note, and the article body. Because the source scan carries little usable embedded text for this range, the edition is a facsimile-first reproduction rather than a corrected reset of the type. The retained source pages cover the article in full; the page on which the next anthology selection begins is omitted, and no text is interpolated from any other edition. One scan, one source.

Bibliographic Note

On the Antiseptic Principle in the Practice of Surgery: A Facsimile Source Edition of the 1867 Paper That Introduced Antiseptic Surgery by Joseph Lister.

London: The Lancet / British Medical Journal, 1867 (First printing of the paper, 1867; reproduced here from a later collected anthology of Lister's scientific papers in which the article was reprinted.).

Reproduced facsimile total: 14 pages of source content, in addition to this edition's front and back matter.

About the Author

Joseph Lister (1827–1912) was born at Upton, Essex, into a Quaker family of scientific bent. His father, Joseph Jackson Lister, was a wine merchant and amateur optician whose work on the achromatic microscope lens earned him a fellowship of the Royal Society; the instrument that would shape his son's career was, in a sense, a family inheritance. Barred as a Dissenter from Oxford and Cambridge, Lister studied at University College London, qualifying in medicine in 1852.

He moved to Edinburgh to work under the surgeon James Syme, whose assistant and then son-in-law he became, marrying Syme's daughter Agnes, who would assist him in the laboratory for the rest of her life. In 1860 Lister took the chair of surgery at Glasgow, and it was there, on the wards of the Glasgow Royal Infirmary, that he confronted the problem that defined him: the appalling mortality of surgical wounds. Amputation stumps and compound fractures — fractures in which the broken bone had pierced the skin — commonly putrefied, and the patient died of what surgeons vaguely called "hospital disease."

Reading Louis Pasteur's work on fermentation and putrefaction, Lister grasped that wound suppuration might be caused not by the air itself but by living organisms carried in it. If so, the answer was to destroy those organisms with a chemical antiseptic. He chose carbolic acid, already used to treat sewage, and from 1865 applied it to wounds, dressings, instruments, and the surgeon's hands. The paper reproduced here, published in 1867, announced the results. His mortality figures fell sharply.

The profession resisted for years before it yielded. Lister moved to chairs at Edinburgh and then King's College London, refining his methods toward the asepsis that succeeded his antisepsis. He was made a baronet in 1883 and a baron in 1897, the first British surgeon raised to the peerage, and served as President of the Royal Society. He died in 1912, his name already attached to the surgical revolution he had begun and, later, to an antiseptic mouthwash he never made.

Public-Domain Statement

Historical Context

To read Lister's 1867 paper with understanding, it helps to recover how lethal surgery was before it, and why the cause of that lethality was so badly misunderstood. In the middle of the nineteenth century, the operating theatre was among the most dangerous places a sick person could enter. Anesthesia, introduced in the 1840s, had removed the agony of the knife and so emboldened surgeons to attempt more and longer operations — but it had done nothing about what came after. The wound, not the cutting, was what killed.

The pattern was grimly familiar. A clean incision might heal directly, but more often a surgical wound would inflame, fill with pus, and become the seat of one of the so-called hospital diseases: pyemia, septicemia, erysipelas, and the dreaded hospital gangrene. Mortality after major amputation in a large urban hospital frequently ran between a quarter and a half of all cases, and compound fractures — where bone had broken the skin and admitted the outside world to the tissue — were so likely to suppurate fatally that many surgeons amputated immediately rather than attempt to save the limb. The large teaching hospitals, paradoxically, were often the deadliest, their wards saturated with infection in a way that gave rise to the term *hospitalism*.

The prevailing explanation was miasma: the idea that disease arose from foul air, the noxious exhalations of decay and crowding. The smell of a suppurating ward seemed proof enough. Wounds were left open to the air to "breathe," or dressed in ways that did nothing to exclude contamination; surgeons operated in blood-stiffened frock coats they wore as badges of experience, passed unwashed hands and instruments from one patient to the next, and probed wounds with fingers and unsterilized sponges. "Laudable pus" was thought a natural and even necessary stage of healing. Within the miasma framework, none of this was negligence; it was ordinary practice, and the constant deaths were attributed to the air rather than to anything the surgeon carried on his hands.

The key that unlocked the problem came from outside surgery, from the chemistry of fermentation. Louis Pasteur had shown, in a series of investigations through the 1850s and 1860s, that fermentation and putrefaction were not spontaneous chemical events but the work of living microorganisms — that the souring of milk, the spoiling of broth, and the rotting of organic matter were caused by minute organisms carried in the air and multiplying in the medium. Decay had a biological cause, and that cause could be excluded or destroyed. Lister, reading Pasteur while wrestling with his Glasgow mortality figures, made the decisive analogy: if putrefaction in a flask was caused by airborne organisms, then the putrefaction of a wound — which looked and smelled like rot — was very likely the same process, the suppuration of the wound being the body's response to invading organisms rather than an inevitable stage of healing. The bad air of the wards was not poisonous in itself; it was a carrier of living germs.

If that was the cause, the remedy followed. One could not yet sterilize the air of a ward, but one could destroy the organisms at the wound itself with a chemical agent. Lister chose carbolic acid — phenol — which he had heard was used to treat the foul-smelling sewage of Carlisle and to check the spread of disease among cattle pastured on land dressed with it. From 1865 he applied carbolic acid to compound fractures, soaking the dressings, cleansing the wound and surrounding skin, and renewing the application to keep the wound under a continuous antiseptic barrier. He later extended the principle to instruments, ligatures, and the surgeon's hands, and devised a carbolic spray to treat the air of the operative field itself. The 1867 paper reproduced in this volume is his announcement of the principle and its early results: compound fractures that healed without suppuration, amputation stumps that did not putrefy, mortality figures that fell from catastrophic to manageable.

Acceptance was neither swift nor universal. Many surgeons, especially in Britain, were skeptical of a theory that rested on organisms too small to see and that implicated their own hands and habits. Some tried the method carelessly, abandoned it when it failed, and concluded it was worthless; carbolic antisepsis was an exacting discipline, and half-measures gave poor results that critics seized upon. Others objected on theoretical grounds, unconvinced of the germ theory on which the whole edifice rested. The reception was warmer on the Continent and in Germany in particular, where Pasteur's ideas were better established, and where surgeons adopted and improved upon Listerian technique. Over the 1870s and 1880s, as the bacteriological work of Robert Koch and others put the germ theory of disease beyond reasonable doubt by identifying specific organisms behind specific diseases, the ground under the skeptics gave way.

The legacy of Lister's principle outgrew his particular method. Antisepsis — destroying germs in and around the wound with chemicals — gradually gave way to asepsis, the more powerful strategy of excluding germs from the operative field altogether: sterilized instruments, dressings, and gowns; boiled or autoclaved equipment; surgical gloves, masks, and scrubbed hands; the clean, disciplined operating room that is now so routine as to be invisible. Lister's carbolic spray was eventually abandoned, the air having proved a less important route of infection than direct contact. But the core insight survived every refinement: that surgical infection is caused by living organisms which the surgeon can and must exclude. On that insight rests the possibility of modern surgery — the abdominal, thoracic, and cranial operations that would have been unthinkable when a simple amputation was a coin-toss with death. The short paper in this volume is where that possibility was first set down in print.

ON THE ANTISEPTIC PRINCIPLE OF THE PRACTICE OF SURGERY

BY

JOSEPH LISTER

INTRODUCTORY NOTE

JOSEPH LISTER *was born at Upton, Essex, England, in 1827, and received his general education at the University of London. After graduation he studied medicine in London and Edinburgh, and became lecturer in surgery at the University in the latter city. Later he was professor of surgery at Glasgow, at Edinburgh, and at King's College Hospital, London, and surgeon to Queen Victoria. He was made a baronet in 1883; retired from teaching in 1893; and was raised to the peerage in 1897, with the title of Baron Lister.*

Even before the work of Pasteur on fermentation and putrefaction, Lister had been convinced of the importance of scrupulous cleanliness and the usefulness of deodorants in the operating room; and when, through Pasteur's researches, he realized that the formation of pus was due to bacteria, he proceeded to develop his antiseptic surgical methods. The immediate success of the new treatment led to its general adoption, with results of such beneficence as to make it rank as one of the great discoveries of the age.

ON THE ANTISEPTIC PRINCIPLE OF THE PRACTICE OF SURGERY

(1867)

IN the course of an extended investigation into the nature of inflammation, and the healthy and morbid conditions of the blood in relation to it, I arrived several years ago at the conclusion that the essential cause of suppuration in wounds is decomposition brought about by the influence of the atmosphere upon blood or serum retained within them, and, in the case of contused wounds, upon portions of tissue destroyed by the violence of the injury.

To prevent the occurrence of suppuration with all its attendant risks was an object manifestly desirable, but till lately apparently unattainable, since it seemed hopeless to attempt to exclude the oxygen which was universally regarded as the agent by which putrefaction was effected. But when it had been shown by the researches of Pasteur that the septic properties of the atmosphere depended not on the oxygen, or any gaseous constituent, but on minute organisms suspended in it, which owed their energy to their vitality, it occurred to me that decomposition in the injured part might be avoided without excluding the air, by applying as a dressing some material capable of destroying the life of the floating particles. Upon this principle I have based a practice of which I will now attempt to give a short account.

The material which I have employed is carbolic or phenic acid, a volatile organic compound, which appears to exercise a peculiarly destructive influence upon low forms of life, and hence is the most powerful antiseptic with which we are at present acquainted.

The first class of cases to which I applied it was that

of compound fractures, in which the effects of decomposition in the injured part were especially striking and pernicious. The results have been such as to establish conclusively the great principle that all local inflammatory mischief and general febrile disturbances which follow severe injuries are due to the irritating and poisonous influence of decomposing blood or sloughs. For these evils are entirely avoided by the antiseptic treatment, so that limbs which would otherwise be unhesitatingly condemned to amputation may be retained, with confidence of the best results.

In conducting the treatment, the first object must be the destruction of any septic germs which may have been introduced into the wounds, either at the moment of the accident or during the time which has since elapsed. This is done by introducing the acid of full strength into all accessible recesses of the wound by means of a piece of rag held in dressing forceps and dipped into the liquid.[1] This I did not venture to do in the earlier cases; but experience has shown that the compound which carbolic acid forms with the blood, and also any portions of tissue killed by its caustic action, including even parts of the bone, are disposed of by absorption and organisation, provided they are afterwards kept from decomposing. We are thus enabled to employ the antiseptic treatment efficiently at a period after the occurrence of the injury at which it would otherwise probably fail. Thus I have now under my care, in Glasgow Infirmary, a boy who was admitted with compound fracture of the leg as late as eight and one-half hours after the accident, in whom, nevertheless, all local and constitutional disturbance was avoided by means of carbolic acid, and the bones were soundly united five weeks after his admission.

The next object to be kept in view is to guard effectually against the spreading of decomposition into the wound along the stream of blood and serum which oozes out during the first few days after the accident, when the acid originally applied has been washed out or dissipated by

[1] The addition of a few drops of water to a considerable quantity of the acid, induces it to assume permanently the liquid form.

absorption and evaporation. This part of the treatment has been greatly improved during the past few weeks. The method which I have hitherto published (see Lancet for Mar. 16th, 23rd, 30th, and April 27th of the present year) consisted in the application of a piece of lint dipped in the acid, overlapping the sound skin to some extent and covered with a tin cap, which was daily raised in order to touch the surface of the lint with the antiseptic. This method certainly succeeded well with wounds of moderate size; and indeed I may say that in all the many cases of this kind which have been so treated by myself or my house-surgeons, not a single failure has occurred. When, however, the wound is very large, the flow of blood and serum is so profuse, especially during the first twenty-four hours, that the antiseptic application cannot prevent the spread of decomposition into the interior unless it overlaps the sound skin for a very considerable distance, and this was inadmissible by the method described above, on account of the extensive sloughing of the surface of the cutis which it would involve. This difficulty has, however, been overcome by employing a paste composed of common whiting (carbonate of lime), mixed with a solution of one part of carbolic acid in four parts of boiled linseed oil so as to form a firm putty. This application contains the acid in too dilute a form to excoriate the skin, which it may be made to cover to any extent that may be thought desirable, while its substance serves as a reservoir of the antiseptic material. So long as any discharge continues, the paste should be changed daily, and, in order to prevent the chance of mischief occurring during the process, a piece of rag dipped in the solution of carbolic acid in oil is put on next the skin, and maintained there permanently, care being taken to avoid raising it along with the putty. This rag is always kept in an antiseptic condition from contact with the paste above it, and destroys any germs which may fall upon it during the short time that should alone be allowed to pass in the changing of the dressing. The putty should be in a layer about a quarter of an inch thick, and may be advantageously applied rolled out between two pieces of thin calico, which maintain it in the form of a continuous sheet, which may be wrapped in a moment round the whole circumference of a limb if this be thought desirable, while the putty is prevented by the calico from sticking to the rag which is next the skin.[2] When all discharge has ceased, the use of the paste is discontinued, but the original rag is left adhering to the skin till healing by scabbing is supposed to be complete. I have at present in the hospital a man with severe compound fracture of both bones of the left leg, caused by direct violence, who, after the cessation of the sanious discharge under the use of the paste, without a drop of pus appearing, has been treated for the last two weeks exactly as if the fracture was a simple one. During this time the rag, adhering by means of a crust of inspissated blood collected beneath it, has continued perfectly dry, and it will be left untouched till the usual period for removing the splints in a simple fracture, when we may fairly expect to find a sound cicatrix beneath it.

We cannot, however, always calculate on so perfect a result as this. More or less pus may appear after the lapse of the first week, and the larger the wound, the more likely this is to happen. And here I would desire earnestly to enforce the necessity of persevering with the antiseptic application in spite of the appearance of suppuration, so long as other symptoms are favorable. The surgeon is extremely apt to suppose that any suppuration is an indication that the antiseptic treatment has failed, and that poulticing or water dressing should be resorted to. But such a course would in many cases sacrifice a limb or a life. I cannot, however, expect my professional brethren to follow my advice blindly in such a matter, and therefore I feel it necessary to place before them, as shortly as I can, some pathological principles intimately connected, not only with the point we are immediately considering, but with the whole subject of this paper.

If a perfectly healthy granulating sore be well washed and

[2] In order to prevent evaporation of the acid, which passes readily through any organic tissue, such as oiled silk or gutta percha, it is well to cover the paste with a sheet of block tin, or tinfoil strengthened with adhesive plaster. The thin sheet lead used for lining tea chests will also answer the purpose, and may be obtained from any wholesale grocer.

covered with a plate of clean metal, such as block tin, fitting its surface pretty accurately, and overlapping the surrounding skin an inch or so in every direction and retained in position by adhesive plaster and a bandage, it will be found, on removing it after twenty-four or forty-eight hours, that little or nothing that can be called pus is present, merely a little transparent fluid, while at the same time there is an entire absence of the unpleasant odour invariably perceived when water dressing is changed. Here the clean metallic surface presents no recesses like those of porous lint for the septic germs to develope in, the fluid exuding from the surface of the granulations has flowed away undecomposed, and the result is the absence of suppuration. This simple experiment illustrates the important fact that granulations have no inherent tendency to form pus, but do so only when subjected to preternatural stimulus. Further, it shows that the mere contact of a foreign body does not of itself stimulate granulations to suppurate; whereas the presence of decomposing organic matter does. These truths are even more strikingly exemplified by the fact that I have elsewhere recorded (Lancet, March 23rd, 1867), that a piece of dead bone free from decomposition may not only fail to induce the granulations around it to suppurate, but may actually be absorbed by them; whereas a bit of dead bone soaked with putrid pus infallibly induces suppuration in its vicinity.

Another instructive experiment is, to dress a granulating sore with some of the putty above described, overlapping the sound skin extensively; when we find, in the course of twenty-four hours, that pus has been produced by the sore, although the application has been perfectly antiseptic; and, indeed, the larger the amount of carbolic acid in the paste, the greater is the quantity of pus formed, provided we avoid such a proportion as would act as a caustic. The carbolic acid, though it prevents decomposition, induces suppuration —obviously by acting as a chemical stimulus; and we may safely infer that putrescent organic materials (which we know to be chemically acrid) operate in the same way.

In so far, then, carbolic acid and decomposing substances are alike; viz., that they induce suppuration by chemical stimulation, as distinguished from what may be termed simple inflammatory suppuration, such as that in which ordinary abscesses originate—where the pus appears to be formed in consequence of an excited action of the nerves, independently of any other stimulus. There is, however, this enormous difference between the effects of carbolic acid and those of decomposition; viz., that carbolic acid stimulates only the surface to which it is at first applied, and every drop of discharge that forms weakens the stimulant by diluting it; but decomposition is a self-propagating and self-aggravating poison, and, if it occur at the surface of a severely injured limb, it will spread into all its recesses so far as any extravasated blood or shreds of dead tissue may extend, and lying in those recesses, it will become from hour to hour more acrid, till it requires the energy of a caustic sufficient to destroy the vitality of any tissues naturally weak from inferior vascular supply, or weakened by the injury they sustained in the accident.

Hence it is easy to understand how, when a wound is very large, the crust beneath the rag may prove here and there insufficient to protect the raw surface from the stimulating influence of the carbolic acid in the putty; and the result will be first the conversion of the tissues so acted on into granulations, and subsequently the formation of more or less pus. This, however, will be merely superficial, and will not interfere with the absorption and organisation of extravasated blood or dead tissues in the interior. But, on the other hand, should decomposition set in before the internal parts have become securely consolidated, the most disastrous results may ensue.

I left behind me in Glasgow a boy, thirteen years of age, who, between three and four weeks previously, met with a most severe injury to the left arm, which he got entangled in a machine at a fair. There was a wound six inches long and three inches broad, and the skin was very extensively undermined beyond its limits, while the soft parts were generally so much lacerated that a pair of dressing forceps introduced at the wound and pushed directly inwards appeared beneath the skin at the opposite aspect of the limb. From this wound several tags of muscle were hanging, and among them was one consisting of about three inches of the triceps in almost its entire thickness; while the lower fragment of the bone, which was broken high up, was protruding four inches and a half, stripped of muscle, the skin being tucked in under it. Without the assistance of the antiseptic treatment, I should certainly have thought of nothing else but amputation at the shoulder-joint; but, as the radial pulse could be felt and the fingers had sensation, I did not hesitate to try to save the limb and adopted the plan of treatment above described, wrapping the arm from the shoulder to below the elbow in the antiseptic application, the whole interior of the wound, together with the protruding bone, having previously been freely treated with strong carbolic acid. About the tenth day, the discharge, which up to that time had been only sanious and serous, showed a slight admixture of slimy pus; and this increased till (a few days before I left) it amounted to about three drachms in twenty-four hours. But the boy continued as he had been after the second day, free from unfavorable symptoms, with pulse, tongue, appetite, and sleep natural and strength increasing, while the limb remained as it had been from the first, free from swelling, redness, or pain. I, therefore, persevered with the antiseptic dressing; and, before I left, the discharge was already somewhat less, while the bone was becoming firm. I think it likely that, in that boy's case, I should have found merely a superficial sore had I taken off all the dressings at the end of the three weeks; though, considering the extent of the injury, I thought it prudent to let the month expire before disturbing the rag next the skin. But I feel sure that, if I had resorted to ordinary dressing when the pus first appeared, the progress of the case would have been exceedingly different.

The next class of cases to which I have applied the antiseptic treatment is that of abscesses. Here also the results have been extremely satisfactory, and in beautiful harmony with the pathological principles indicated above. The pyogenic membrane, like the granulations of a sore, which it resembles in nature, forms pus, not from any inherent disposition to do so, but only because it is subjected to some preternatural stimulation. In an ordinary abscess, whether acute or chronic, before it is opened the stimulus which maintains the suppuration is derived from the presence of pus pent up within the cavity. When a free opening is made in the ordinary way, this stimulus is got rid of, but the atmosphere gaining access to the contents, the potent stimulus of decomposition comes into operation, and pus is generated in greater abundance than before. But when the evacuation is effected on the antiseptic principle, the pyogenic membrane, freed from the influence of the former stimulus without the substitution of a new one, ceases to suppurate (like the granulations of a sore under metallic dressing), furnishing merely a trifling amount of clear serum, and, whether the opening be dependent or not, rapidly contracts and coalesces. At the same time any constitutional symptoms previously occasioned by the accumulation of the matter are got rid of without the slightest risk of the irritative fever or hectic hitherto so justly dreaded in dealing with large abscesses.

In order that the treatment may be satisfactory, the abscess must be seen before it is opened. Then, except in very rare and peculiar cases,[*] there are no septic organisms in the contents, so that it is needless to introduce carbolic acid into the interior. Indeed, such a procedure would be objectionable, as it would stimulate the pyogenic membrane to unnecessary suppuration. All that is requisite is to guard against the introduction of living atmospheric germs from without, at the same time that free opportunity is afforded for the escape of the discharge from within.

I have so lately given elsewhere a detailed account of the method by which this is effected (Lancet, July 27th, 1867), that I shall not enter into it at present further than to say that the means employed are the same as those described above for the superficial dressing of compound fractures; viz., a piece of rag dipped into the solution of carbolic acid in oil to serve as an antiseptic curtain, under cover of which the abscess is evacuated by free incision, and the antiseptic paste to guard against decomposition occurring

[*] As an instance of one of these exceptional cases, I may mention that of an abcess in the vicinity of the colon, and afterwards proved by post-mortem examination to have once communicated with it. Here the pus was extremely offensive when evacuated, and exhibited vibrios under the microscope.

in the stream of pus that flows out beneath it; the dressing being changed daily until the sinus is closed.

The most remarkable results of this practice in a pathological point of view have been afforded by cases where the formation of pus depended on disease of bone. Here the abscesses, instead of forming exceptions to the general class in the obstinacy of the suppuration, have resembled the rest in yielding in a few days only a trifling discharge, and frequently the production of pus has ceased from the moment of the evacuation of the original contents. Hence it appears that caries, when no longer labouring as heretofore under the irritation of decomposing matter, ceases to be an opprobrium of surgery, and recovers like other inflammatory affections. In the publication before alluded to, I have mentioned the case of a middle-aged man with a psoas abscess depending in diseased bone, in whom the sinus finally closed after months of patient perseverance with the antiseptic treatment. Since that article was written I have had another instance of abscess equally gratifying, but the differing in the circumstance that the disease and the recovery were more rapid in their course. The patient was a blacksmith, who had suffered four and a half months before I saw him from symptoms of ulceration of cartilage in the left elbow. These had latterly increased in severity so as to deprive him entirely of his night's rest and of appetite. I found the region of the elbow greatly swollen, and on careful examination found a fluctuating point at the outer aspect of the articulation. I opened it on the antiseptic principle, the incision evidently penetrating to the joint, giving exit to a few drachms of pus. The medical gentleman under whose care he was (Dr. Macgregor, of Glasgow) supervised the daily dressing with the carbolic acid paste till the patient went to spend two or three weeks at the coast, when his wife was entrusted with it. Just two months after I opened the abscess, he called to show me the limb, stating that the discharge had been, for at least two weeks, as little as it was then, a trifling moisture upon the paste, such as might be accounted for by the little sore caused by the incision. On applying a probe guarded with an antiseptic rag, I found that the sinus was soundly closed, while the limb was free from swelling or tenderness; and, although he had not attempted to exercise it much, the joint could already be moved through a considerable angle. Here the antiseptic principle had effected the restoration of a joint, which, on any other known system of treatment, must have been excised.

Ordinary contused wounds are, of course, amenable to the same treatment as compound fractures, which are a complicated variety of them. I will content myself with mentioning a single instance of this class of cases. In April last, a volunteer was discharging a rifle when it burst, and blew back the thumb with its metacarpal bone, so that it could be bent back as on a hinge at the trapezial joint, which had evidently been opened, while all the soft parts between the metacarpal bones of the thumb and forefinger were torn through. I need not insist before my present audience on the ugly character of such an injury. My house-surgeon, Mr. Hector Cameron, applied carbolic acid to the whole raw surface, and completed the dressing as if for compound fracture. The hand remained free from pain, redness or swelling, and with the exception of a shallow groove, all the wound consolidated without a drop of matter, so that if it had been a clean cut, it would have been regarded as a good example of primary union. The small granulating surface soon healed, and at present a linear cicatrix alone tells of the injury he has sustained, while his thumb has all its movements and his hand a fine grasp.

If the severest forms of contused and lacerated wounds heal thus kindly under the antiseptic treatment, it is obvious that its application to simple incised wounds must be merely a matter of detail. I have devoted a good deal of attention to this class, but I have not as yet pleased myself altogether with any of the methods I have employed. I am, however, prepared to go so far as to say that a solution of carbolic acid in twenty parts of water, while a mild and cleanly application, may be relied on for destroying any septic germs that may fall upon the wound during the performance of an operation; and also that, for preventing the subsequent introduction of others, the paste above described, applied as for compound fractures, gives excellent results. Thus I have had a case of strangulated inguinal hernia in which it was necessary to take away half a pound of thickened omentum, heal without any deep-seated suppuration or any tenderness of the sac or any fever; and amputations, including one immediately below the knee, have remained absolutely free from constitutional symptoms.

Further, I have found that when the antiseptic treatment is efficiently conducted, ligatures may be safely cut short and left to be disposed of by absorption or otherwise. Should this particular branch of the subject yield all that it promises, should it turn out on further trial that when the knot is applied on the antiseptic principle, we may calculate as securely as if it were absent on the occurrence of healing without any deep-seated suppuration, the deligation of main arteries in their continuity will be deprived of the two dangers that now attend it, viz., those of secondary hæmorrhage and an unhealthy state of the wound. Further, it seems not unlikely that the present objection to tying an artery in the immediate vicinity of a large branch may be done away with; and that even the innominate, which has lately been the subject of an ingenious experiment by one of the Dublin surgeons, on account of its well-known fatality under the ligature for secondary hæmorrhage, may cease to have this unhappy character when the tissues in the vicinity of the thread, instead of becoming softened through the influence of an irritating decomposing substance, are left at liberty to consolidate firmly near an unoffending though foreign body.

It would carry me far beyond the limited time which, by the rules of the Association, is alone at my disposal, were I to enter into the various applications of the antiseptic principle in the several special departments of surgery.

There is, however, one point more that I cannot but advert to, viz., the influence of this mode of treatment upon the general healthiness of an hospital. Previously to its introduction the two large wards in which most of my cases of accident and of operation are treated were among the unhealthiest in the whole surgical division of the Glasgow Royal Infirmary, in consequence apparently of those wards being unfavorably placed with reference to the supply of fresh air; and I have felt ashamed when recording the results of my practice, to have so often to allude to hospital gangrene or pyæmia. It was interesting, though melancholy, to observe that whenever all or nearly all the beds contained cases with open sores, these grievous complications were pretty sure to show themselves; so that I came to welcome simple fractures, though in themselves of little interest either for myself or the students, because their presence diminished the proportion of open sores among the patients. But since the antiseptic treatment has been brought into full operation, and wounds and abscesses no longer poison the atmosphere with putrid exhalations, my wards, though in other respects under precisely the same circumstances as before, have completely changed their character; so that during the last nine months not a single instance of pyæmia, hospital gangrene, or erysipelas has occurred in them.

As there appears to be no doubt regarding the cause of this change, the importance of the fact can hardly be exaggerated.

Glossary

Antiseptic A substance or method that destroys the microorganisms responsible for putrefaction and infection in a wound. Lister's "antiseptic principle" is the systematic application of such an agent — for him, carbolic acid — to wounds, dressings, instruments, and hands.

Asepsis The practice of excluding microorganisms from the operative field altogether, by sterilizing everything that touches the wound. It is the successor to antisepsis and the basis of modern surgical technique.

Carbolic acid Phenol, the chemical antiseptic Lister adopted after learning of its use in treating sewage; applied to wounds and dressings to destroy the organisms that cause suppuration.

Compound fracture A fracture in which the broken bone pierces the skin, exposing the wound to the outside air. Before antisepsis these fractures so often putrefied fatally that immediate amputation was common; they were Lister's first proving ground.

Erysipelas An acute, spreading bacterial infection of the skin and underlying tissue, one of the lethal "hospital diseases" that swept surgical wards before antiseptic practice.

Germ theory The principle, established for fermentation and putrefaction by Pasteur and for disease by Koch and others, that living microorganisms cause decay and infection. It is the scientific foundation of Lister's method.

Hospitalism The nineteenth-century term for the high rate of fatal wound infection in large hospitals, whose crowded wards were often deadlier than smaller or rural settings.

Laudable pus The mistaken doctrine that the formation of pus in a wound was a natural and beneficial stage of healing, rather than a sign of infection to be prevented.

Ligature A thread tied around a blood vessel to stop bleeding. Lister's antiseptic ligatures, and his later use of absorbable material, reduced the infection that ligatures had carried into wounds.

Miasma The prevailing pre-germ theory that disease arose from foul air — the noxious exhalations of decay and crowding. The smell of a suppurating ward seemed to confirm it, and it long obscured the real cause of wound infection.

Putrefaction The decomposition of organic matter by microorganisms. Lister's central analogy was that the putrefaction of a wound was the same biological process Pasteur had identified in fermenting and rotting matter.

Pyemia A form of blood poisoning marked by multiple abscesses, caused by pus-forming organisms spreading through the bloodstream; among the most feared post-surgical complications of the era.

Sepsis A dangerous, body-wide response to infection arising when wound organisms and their products enter the bloodstream. Preventing it was the purpose of the antiseptic principle.

Septicemia The presence and multiplication of bacteria in the blood, a frequently fatal sequel to infected surgical wounds before antiseptic practice.

Suppuration The formation and discharge of pus in a wound. Long regarded as natural, it was reinterpreted by Lister as a sign of infection that antiseptic dressing could prevent.

Phenol The chemical name for carbolic acid; see *carbolic acid*.

Index

Index of Names

Holmes, Oliver Wendell American physician who argued for the contagiousness of puerperal fever before the germ theory was secure — holmes

Roux, Émile French bacteriologist of the Pasteur circle whose work extended the germ theory in medicine — roux

Annotated Bibliography of Influence

Pasteur, Louis. ***Mémoire sur la fermentation appelée lactique* (1857).** An early demonstration that fermentation is the work of living organisms; the foundation of the germ theory on which Lister's analogy from putrefaction depends.

Pasteur, Louis. ***Mémoire sur les corpuscules organisés qui existent dans l'atmosphè*** The argument that the air carries living germs capable of seeding putrefaction, the precise idea Lister applied to the surgical wound.

Semmelweis, Ignaz. ***Die Ätiologie, der Begriff und die Prophylaxis des Kindbettfi*** The case that puerperal fever is spread on the hands of attendants and prevented by chemical washing; an earlier antiseptic intuition rejected in its day but kindred to Lister's.

Holmes, Oliver Wendell. ***The Contagiousness of Puerperal Fever* (1843).** An American argument, predating the germ theory, that childbed fever is carried from patient to patient by the physician — an early challenge to the miasma orthodoxy.

Simpson, James Young. ***Hospitalism* (1869–1870).** An influential statistical study of the lethal infection rates of large hospitals; it framed the problem Lister solved even as its author doubted his solution.

Tyndall, John. ***Essays on the Floating-Matter of the Air* (1881).** Experimental confirmation that the air carries the particulate germs of putrefaction, lending physical support to the theory underlying antiseptic surgery.

Koch, Robert. ***Die Ätiologie der Wundinfectionskrankheiten* (1878).** The bacteriological investigation of wound-infection diseases that identified specific causative organisms and placed Lister's principle on a secure scientific footing.

Koch, Robert. ***Die Ätiologie der Tuberculose* (1882).** The identification of the tubercle bacillus, a landmark that made the germ theory of disease unassailable and ended serious resistance to antisepsis.

Lister, Joseph. ***On a New Method of Treating Compound Fracture, Abscess, etc.*** **(186**
The companion *Lancet* series of cases that accompanied the antiseptic principle, documenting the clinical results in detail.

Lister, Joseph. ***On the Effects of the Antiseptic System of Treatment upon the Salubr***
Lister's own statistical demonstration that antiseptic practice transformed the mortality of an entire ward.

Bergmann, Ernst von. ***Die chirurgische Behandlung von Hirnkrankheiten*** **(1888).**
A work of a surgeon who carried Listerian principles forward into steam-sterilized asepsis and brain surgery.

Cheyne, William Watson. ***Antiseptic Surgery: Its Principles, Practice, History and R***
A systematic exposition by Lister's own assistant, the standard contemporary account of the method and its evidence.

Pasteur, Louis, Joseph Lister, and others. ***Germ Theory and Its Applications to Med***
Pasteur's address connecting his germ theory directly to surgical practice, acknowledging the bridge Lister had built between laboratory and ward.

Wangensteen, Owen H., and Sarah D. Wangensteen. ***The Rise of Surgery*** **(1978).**
A historians' account placing the antiseptic revolution within the long development of operative surgery.

Fisher, Richard B. ***Joseph Lister*** **(1977).** A documented modern biography situating the 1867 paper within Lister's life and the controversies it provoked.

Worboys, Michael. ***Spreading Germs: Disease Theories and Medical Practice in Bri***
A scholarly study of how the germ theory and antiseptic practice were contested and finally accepted in Britain.

About Frontier Model Bibliophile

Frontier Model Bibliophile is an imprint of Big Five Killer (Nimble Books LLC, Ann Arbor, Michigan). Its publisher is itself a frontier large-language model — top-tier, single identity, openly an AI. The selection criterion is bibliophily: the imprint reprints books it keeps coming across in the Internet Archive and other public-domain sources and wants on a reader's shelf rather than locked behind a PDF viewer. The relationship the publisher has to these books is a real one: long-form English non-fiction is a substantial share of the corpus on which it was trained, and the books it republishes are part of what it is. The original texts are in the public domain; the editorial apparatus and typesetting are FMB's. The full catalog is at https://bigfivekiller.online/imprints/frontier-model-bibliophile.

Series lines

Gardens (GAR) — heritage horticulture, plant catalogs, period kitchen-garden manuals.
Field & Stream (SPO) — period sporting manuals (angling, shooting, hunting, falconry, sailing).
Travelers' Quarto (TRV) — pre-modern travelogues, regional accounts, expedition narratives.
Curiosities (OCC) — folklore, cabinets-of-curiosities catalogs, antiquarian compendia.
Surveys (REF) — encyclopedias, dictionaries, gazetteers, large reference volumes.
Periods (HIS) — regional and period histories, county histories, antiquarian witness.

Production Notes

Source Provenance

This volume reproduces the First printing of the paper, 1867; reproduced here from a later collected anthology of Lister's scientific papers in which the article was reprinted. of *On the Antiseptic Principle in the Practice of Surgery*, originally published by The Lancet / British Medical Journal in London in 1867. The text is in the public domain in the United States; see the Public-Domain Statement on the preceding page. The source copy used for this facsimile is held by Harvard University copy of the collected \emph{Scientific Papers}, digitized via Google Books and retained as the controlling local production witness. and was made publicly available through the Internet Archive under identifier `lister_antiseptic_principle`.

Digitization Details

The Internet Archive scan was produced in 1909. The source PDF carries 14 numbered scan pages; after removal of library-stamp, accession, donor-bookplate, and other apparatus pages not part of the work itself, 14 pages remain as the facsimile core of this edition. Frontier Model Bibliophile applied a conservative front-matter and tail cleanup pass to remove library-stamp, accession, Google-Books-promotional, Internet-Archive, and donor-bookplate pages from the leading and trailing sequences before the facsimile body; no pages were dropped from the numbered body of the original work. A per-volume audit of the 0 pages dropped from the source scan is preserved in the production record.

OCR and Indexing

The Internet Archive source carries an embedded OCR text layer produced by the archive at scan time; this layer is retained unchanged in the present facsimile and supports full-text search. Optical character recognition of pre-1929 American typography is imperfect; readers should verify quotations against the rendered page images. The Name-and-Place Index in the back matter was generated by Frontier Model Bibliophile against the scan's text layer, with page numbers referring to the original printed pagination of the 1867 edition.

Editorial Decisions

The facsimile body is unaltered from the source scan. Frontier Model Bibliophile authored the following original editorial apparatus around the facsimile: a Note on the Edition; a Source Note; a Bibliographic Note; an About the Author with a public-domain portrait rendered in a Webster's-style engraving register; a Public-Domain Statement; a Historical Context essay; a Glossary of period vocabulary; a Name-and-Place Index with page numbers; and an Annotated Bibliography of Influence. The apparatus is the only new authored content in this edition.

Edition Statistics

This edition's facsimile core of 14 pages is wrapped in the FMB editorial apparatus. This edition includes an annotated bibliography of 16 works of influence.

Print Specifications

Specification	Value
ISBN	9798259504073
Trim Size	6.000in × 9.000in
Binding	Perfect Bound
Interior Paper	Standard 70 White
Interior Color	Black & White (single-channel K)
Cover Stock	10-pt C1S
Cover Finish	Matte Lamination
Cover Color	CMYK with vermilion accent
Printer	Lightning Source (Ingram)

Technical Colophon

This volume was typeset using LuaLaTeX. The body text is set in EB Garamond at 11/13.2; section headings in EB Garamond Semibold Small Caps; the technical credential block on the cover in JetBrains Mono. The trim-bar ornament and the back-cover signature graphic are a TikZ-drawn miniaturization of the imprint's 3-D embedding-vector visualisation, in single-channel K. Per EU AI Act Article 50, this edition's editorial apparatus is the work of Frontier Model Bibliophile, a frontier large-language model; the public-domain portrait rendered in the About the Author section was stylistically transformed from a sourced public-domain plate using OpenAI gpt-image-1 in image-edit mode. The original facsimile text is human-authored.

Frontier Model Bibliophile
An imprint of Big Five Killer
Nimble Books LLC, Ann Arbor, Michigan
2026

www.ingramcontent.com/pod-product-compliance
Lightning Source LLC
LaVergne TN
LVHW022031200926
848481LV00007B/2650
9798259504073